The Apple Cider Vinegar Weight Loss Diet

Melody McAdams

DEDICATION

This book is dedicated to my research partner and husband, Jay. We have been a proponent of healthy living it seems like forever. I couldn't have done it without his tireless effort in helping put this all together.

ACKNOWLEDGMENTS

I would like to give much credit to my editor and friend, Helen Parker. She worked with me getting this to paper. To Bruce and Millie for helping take care of the kids during the last few chapters. Lastly, but not least, my husband, Jay for helping so much on the research of this book.

Contents

Introduction

Weight loss can feel like an uphill battle for the millions of Americans who are struggling to regain their health and figure. Unsurprisingly, weight loss has turned into a billion-dollar industry – there are diet books, exercise tapes, video games, pills, herbal supplements, fitness equipment and weight loss consultation services available for purchase, and a desperate individual may throw thousands of dollars at these products to see only minimal results. Long-term success rates are low, and frustrated dieters often find themselves caught in a state of "yo-yo dieting"; they're stuck in an endless (and harmful) loop of losing and re-gaining weight.

It's not all doom and gloom for an overweight individual, however. There are perfectly safe and effective methods for weight loss that require no more than a trip to the grocery store – no pills, no surgeries and no gimmicks. In fact, there is one weight-loss superstar that you've probably browsed right past at the grocery store: Apple Cider Vinegar. This eBook will teach you how to use apple cider vinegar to craft a healthier lifestyle and new, slimmer body for yourself, at minimal cost and effort.

Always remember that safe, permanent weight loss is possible. All you'll need is some determination, patience and a little bit of vinegar.

.

1 The Benefits of Apple Cider Vinegar

You've probably seen apple cider vinegar in your local grocery store. You might have picked some up, or you may have strolled right past it, paying it no mind. What is it, anyway? Well, as you have suspected, apple cider vinegar comes from apple cider. The cider is fermented into alcohol, and the alcohol is allowed to continue fermenting until it becomes vinegar. All vinegar is made this way; if you allowed the wine in your cupboard to continue fermenting, eventually, you'd have vinegar. For hundreds of years, apple cider vinegar has been prescribed as a folk remedy to cure all kinds of ailments – some legitimate cures, some not – and with the resurgence of natural medicine in recent years, the vinegar has found itself back in the health spotlight.

So, what can this incredible vinegar do for you? In a world of rising obesity rates, the most prized property of apple cider vinegar is its ability to suppress appetite. In 2005, a study published in the European Journal of Clinical Nutrition found a direct correlation between the amount of vinegar consumed and the potency of appetite suppression. Subjects in the study were given a piece of bread what was either plain, or soaked with a low, medium, or high amount of vinegar. Subjects who ate the most vinegar reported feeling fullest and most satisfied. Even if you're not a fan of bread, the effect still holds; you can drink the vinegar by itself and feel the same effects.

In other medical circles, apple cider vinegar is prized for an entirely different reason – it's proven to lower blood sugar. This is the most well-researched application of apple cider vinegar. One 2007 study showed that type 2 diabetics (without insulin injections) who took just two tablespoons of vinegar before hitting the sack were found to have much more stable levels of blood glucose in the morning. If you suffer from type 2 diabetes, pre-diabetes or weight-related insulin resistance, apple cider vinegar is an affordable, all-natural treatment that is almost certain to improve your health.

Preliminary animal studies have also found that the vinegar can lower cholesterol and ease high blood pressure. It's not yet known whether these same effects will be found in humans, but scientists believe that some benefit is likely. One study has shown that people who eat vinegar-based salad dressing at least five times per week were at a significantly decreased risk of heart disease. Further study will be needed to pinpoint the exact relationship between apple cider vinegar and heart disease, but these early results are extremely promising.

Another exciting medical property of apple cider vinegar is its potential ability to fight cancer cells. Some studies have shown that vinegar may slow cancer cell growth, or even kill the cells outright. An observational study of humans who regularly took apple cider vinegar found that regular consumption of the vinegar may lead to a decrease in esophageal cancers. These results are only early explorations of the relationship between cancer risk and apple cider vinegar, but once again, the results are promising.

All good things do have a downside, and the downside of apple cider vinegar is its acidity. People taking apple cider vinegar on a regular basis should take steps to protect their teeth. Regular flossing and brushing with a soft-bristled toothbrush is a must, and diluting the vinegar with water or oil may also help to reduce the dangers to tooth enamel. People with acid reflux damage to their esophagus should also use caution when taking apple cider vinegar, as the acid may irritate the damage. The vinegar is available as a supplement, but these tablets are not FDA regulated, and it may be impossible to determine how much vinegar is in each pill.

Insulin-dependent diabetics should also use caution when taking apple cider vinegar, as the drop in blood sugar may require adjustments to their insulin doses. If you have diabetes and take insulin injections, speak to your doctor before starting on an apple cider vinegar weight loss plan.

2 Tracking Calories

Taking advantage of the natural appetite-suppressing properties of apple cider vinegar is certainly an excellent start to your weight loss journey, but it's only a start. The only way to make sure that your weight goes down is to ensure that you consume fewer calories than you need to maintain your current size. Using an appetite suppressant will certainly make this easier, but it's easy to think that using apple cider vinegar in your diet will guarantee results – the only way to be certain that you'll meet your goals is to count calories.

Now, counting your calories may sound tedious and difficult. You're required to measure and write down every morsel of food that goes into your mouth – it can sound like an impossible task. There's no need to worry. Tracking your calories soon becomes second nature, and you'll come to have a much better understanding of nutrition.

Before you can start tracking calories, there are a few things you may need to get. First and foremost, you'll need somewhere to write down your calorie counts. If you're a pen-and-paper sort of person, get yourself a blank notebook; writing things down on scraps of paper will only leave you disorganized and jumbled. Smartphone and tablet users have a variety of free calorie-counting apps at their disposal; some, like the popular 'MyFitnessPal', include free barcode scanning functions that allow you to instantly upload the nutritional information of packaged foods. If your laptop is never far from your hand, you can also use free online calorie tracking websites and diaries, including the companion website to the 'MyFitnessPal' app. There are a few advantages to going high-tech; using calorie-tracking apps is faster and more convenient, and they allow you to effortlessly keep track of not only calories, but fat, saturated fat, sodium, fiber and protein. This extra information is tough to keep track of manually, and it will help you to choose healthy foods.

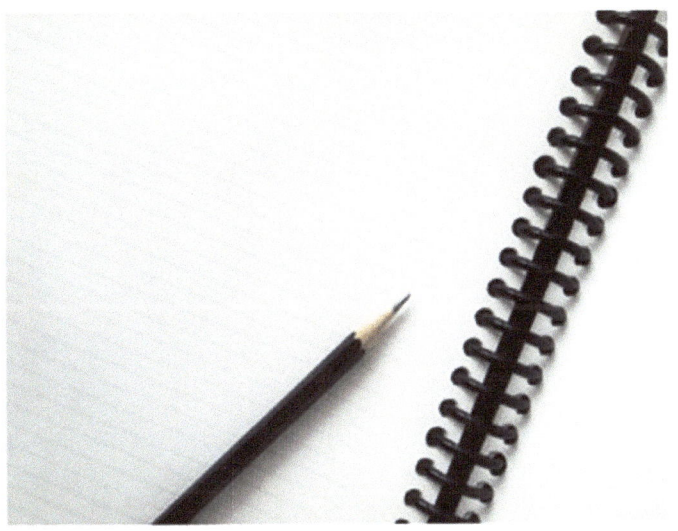

Make sure your notebook pages are wide enough to fit all of your food information.

You should also invest in a food scale – these scales, sometimes called "nutrition scales", are sold in most house wares stores. A mid-range scale will cost roughly $20, but (besides apple cider vinegar) it might be the most valuable dietary aid you ever purchase. A food scale takes the guesswork out of serving sizes.

What does a three-ounce serving of meat look like? What's the difference between a medium- and a large-sized apple? A food scale allows you to find out in seconds, preventing accidental overeating. High-end food scales even offer pre-programmed selections of different types of foods, allowing you to directly measure food by calories instead of weight.

If you plan on manually tracking your calories by hand, you'll also need to find a source of nutritional information. Packaged foods are easy to track, but items like fruits, vegetables and home-baked bread don't come with information labels. If you need to know how many calories are in the pear you just ate, you can turn to one of two places to find out: you can look it up online (a simple Google search will do) or you can get yourself a nutrition reference book. These books – which can be found at any major bookstore – simply list the nutritional information for serving sizes of thousands of common food items. If you're going to be away from internet access for long periods of time, these books are absolutely indispensable.

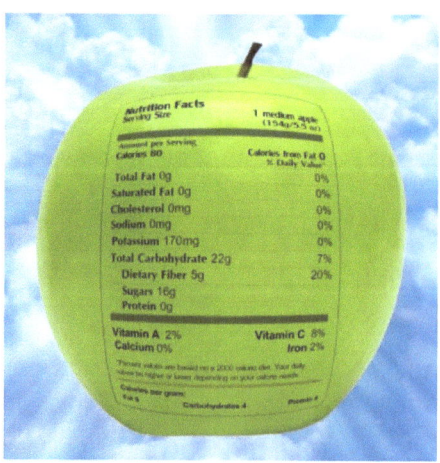

Calorie counting would be much easier if all food came printed

with labels.

Another thing no calorie-conscious person should be without? Tupperware. If you're trying to lose weight and keep it off, you can never have enough of the stuff. Most children in the western world were raised on a "clean your plate" mentality. With all those starving children in Africa to consider, most of us who grew up in developed countries treat wasting food as a cardinal sin; for many people, that very attitude is what led to weight gain in the first place. It's tough to leave that extra half-cup of mashed potato or piece of chicken to go to waste, and many people would sooner polish off the leftovers than see them go into the trash. Tupperware is the solution. No leftover is too small to be stored, which means you can strictly adhere to proper portion sizes. Plus, keeping a collection of stored leftovers is great for sticking to healthy foods – it saves you prep time when you're in a rush, and it helps you control your portions.

Once you're equipped for effective calorie counting, you'll need to set yourself a daily calorie goal. In order to lose weight, you must eat fewer calories than what is needed to maintain your current size. The number of calories you burn just by existing each day is called your "metabolic rate", and there are a few ways to calculate it. The easiest way to find out is to ask your doctor – he or she can give you an accurate estimate and help you set a realistic daily calorie goal. Reliable online calculators (particularly the one offered by webMD) are also a great way to get an estimate. On average, a woman's metabolic rate will fall somewhere around 2000 calories and a man's will fall near 2500.

To lose a single pound in a week, the number of calories you've burned that week must exceed the number of calories you've eaten by 3600. Needless to say, the larger the gap you set between your metabolic rate and your daily calorie intake, the faster you'll lose weight. Now, that's not to say you should go to extremes. Eating fewer than 1200 calories per day will make your body think that you're living through some kind of famine, and, in response, your body will shut down your metabolism to go into a "starvation mode" that conserves precious calories. It seems counter-intuitive, but you do need to eat a minimum amount of food to keep your weight loss from slowing down. Apple cider vinegar should be used to prevent you from overeating, but you should never try to use it to starve yourself.

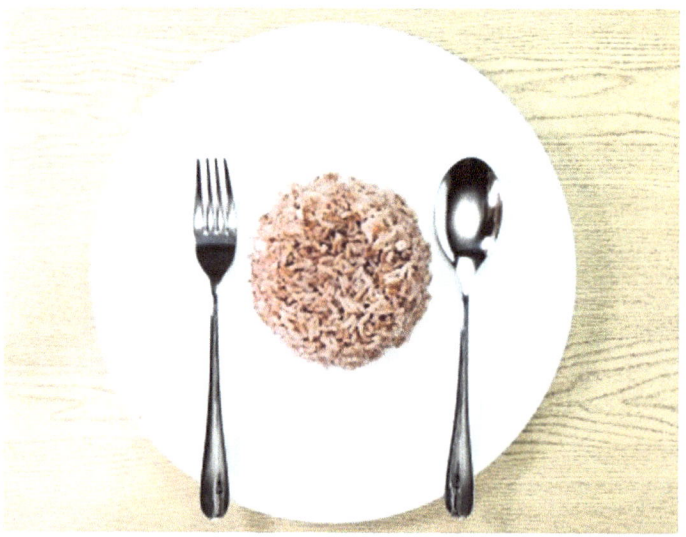

There's a fine line between 'enough' food and 'too little' food.

One of the key reasons that regular calorie counting leads to far greater success than pre-planned diets is that calorie counting places no restrictions on what sorts of foods you can eat. It's human nature to fight restrictions; if you promised yourself that you'd never eat chips again, it's a safe bet that you'll find yourself wolfing down Doritos by the end of the week. If cheesecake is your absolute favorite dessert, you're not going to go the rest of your life without ever tasting it again – that's just not realistic. By combining the use of apple cider vinegar and calorie counting, you can eat small, reasonable portions of your favorite foods and still lose weight. Eating healthy isn't about ceasing to eat cookies; it's about eating fewer of them, less often.

3 Incorporating Exercise

It's tough to find time to exercise these days – you have approximately seven hundred and fourteen things that were supposed to be done yesterday, never mind today's workload. Gym memberships cost more than car payments, and they're so crowded during peak hours. There's no room in the basement for any gym equipment. You're so out of shape, you don't even know where to begin an exercise routine. There are hundreds of excuses for not incorporating exercise into your lifestyle, but no excuse can negate the body's need for activity.

Most of the benefits of exercise are obvious. You've heard them before. You'll have more energy, more endurance, and fewer heart attacks. There are, however, a few extra perks to an active lifestyle that you may not have realized.

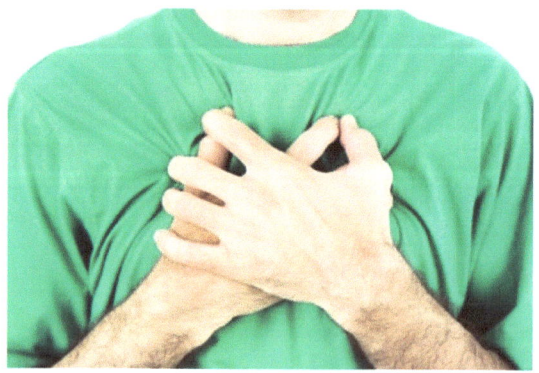

An exercise plan can help you escape an early heart attack.

One of the major concerns with excess weight is the development of insulin resistance and type 2 diabetes. As we previously discussed, apple cider vinegar can help to regulate blood sugar levels, and taking up regular exercise in conjunction with vinegar can really help to reduce problems. Active muscles burn more glucose for energy, which reduces your need for insulin, and aerobic exercise also increases the efficiency of the insulin already in your blood. Over the long term, regular exercise can reduce dangerous high blood sugar and stave off – or even reverse – adult diabetes.

Even those who aren't at risk of developing diabetes can improve their overall heath with added exercise. Every cell in the human body contains a copy of the individual's DNA – DNA being the genetic "instructions", so to speak, for creating that person. In your body, DNA exists as a coil of sugar, and at the end of that coil, there's a 'cap', called a telomere, which prevents DNA from unraveling. As we age, our telomeres get shorter. Eventually, our DNA begins to fray and mutate, leading to problems like age-related symptoms, osteoporosis, and cancer. Luckily, there is a solution. For unknown reasons, exercise slows and even reverses this telomere shortening. Don't think you're too old to start, either – you can improve your genetic health whether you begin exercising at 18 or 80.

The cosmetic benefits of exercise also go beyond the obvious toned muscles. Humans are incredibly adaptable. As you gained weight, your skin stretched to accommodate the extra bulk. As you lose weight, your skin will shrink again, but it may shrink more slowly than you do. People who have lost significant amounts of weight often complain of loose skin, particularly on their stomach and upper arms. It's unattractive and embarrassing, and it doesn't feel like much can be done about it. This loose skin is often still attached to layers of fat beneath the skin; if you exercise frequently, you'll burn that fat and tone muscle, firming your skin in the process.

So you understand the benefits of exercise, but how are you supposed to ease yourself into fitness after months or years of inactivity? It's easy. All you need to do is walk. Walking is aerobic and, unlike running, it doesn't place a lot of strain on your joints. You don't need any special equipment – beyond a good pair of shoes – and you can do it just about anywhere. If the weather permits, you can walk outdoors, but in bad weather, you'll get just as much benefit from walking indoors in your local mall. Try to build up your endurance, walking farther and faster each day, until you can go long distances without feeling tired.

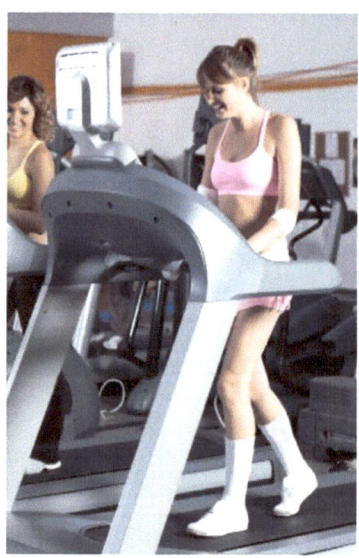

Treadmills are also an option for walking when the weather is poor.

Once you've built up your endurance through walking, you can gradually build up into running. Alternate between walking and running, changing the proportions as you get fitter. You could use lampposts or sidewalk sections to measure your distance – you could run past one lamppost and walk past the next three. Apps like the "Couch to 5K running" app gradually take you from a running novice to an expert. There are books and websites that teach you how to go about it safely, or you could speak to a local running groups for advice.

Another great exercise for beginners is one that overweight people feel the most uncomfortable about – swimming. If you can get over the anxiety of being seen in a bathing suit, swimming is a wonderful choice for someone trying to get in shape. It offers resistance training for every part of your body, while simultaneously offering aerobic exercise. Since you're not supporting your full body weight in the water, there's no risk of strain on your joints. Some public swimming pools even offer aquatic exercise classes that maximize the fitness benefits of swimming.

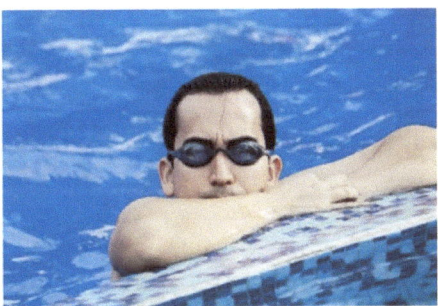

Some pools have special lanes for swimming lengths of the pool.

Biking is another way to easily improve your fitness. As I've mentioned, it's important for beginners to avoid placing undue strain on their joints – especially if they're on the heavy side – and biking offers all the aerobic benefits of running without the pounding pressure on the knees. It also builds leg strength, as you work your quadriceps to propel your body forward.

If you know you'll have a hard time sticking to any kind of regular exercise, consider teaming up with a 'gym buddy'. A bit of friendly competition and support is plenty of motivation to stay active; you don't want to disappoint your friend, do you? Choosing someone who is close to your fitness level means you won't have to be ashamed of yourself; choosing someone slightly more fit than you might be a good way to get some exercise pointers. Commit to a regular schedule, and hold your partner accountable.

If you've got the time and money, it may be worthwhile to invest in exercise classes, or even a personal trainer. These will force you to stick to a schedule and be accountable. A personal trainer will even tailor sessions to your specific fitness level and help you to meet your goals in a realistic time period. If there's a specific fitness event you're training for – like a half-marathon – a personal trainer will help you to get there without injuring yourself.

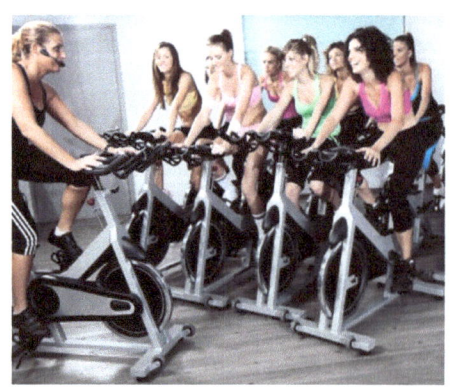

Exercise classes exist for people at all skill levels.

Ultimately, what matters is that you get up and get moving. There's an expression in weight loss that goes "no matter how slowly you go, you're still lapping everyone on the couch"; nothing could be truer. Don't be ashamed of making a slow start – so long as you stick with it, you'll be running circles around your former self in no time.

4 Navigating Temptation

If all of a person's eating took place in a calm, controlled environment filled with healthy options, no one would ever have a weight problem. Unfortunately, the real world doesn't work like that. There are temptations everywhere – on TV, at the grocery store, in restaurants, at parties, and at the office. At times, it can feel like the entire world is involved in a giant conspiracy to keep you in plus-sized pants. So how do you overcome these daily trials and come out with your diet intact? There are a few easy tips you can try.

Never go grocery shopping while hungry. It's impossible to snack on junk food if you don't buy any, which means you need to be at your strongest while you're in the supermarket. When you're ravenous, you're more inclined to think those cakes, cookies, chips, pies, and chocolate bars are a good idea; if you do your grocery shopping when you're full, you'll be prone to head for the fruits and vegetables. Eat a filling meal before embarking on your grocery shopping trip, and be sure to take apple cider vinegar with your meal to prevent any hunger pangs from returning. You'll thank yourself for it later.

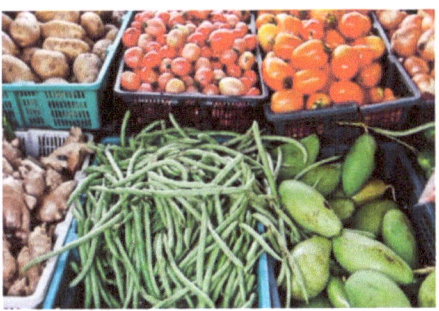

Healthy foods tend to be around the perimeter of the grocery store and not in the aisles.

Look up restaurant menus ahead of time. Your weight loss process shouldn't keep you a prisoner in your own home – you should be able to go out and enjoy yourself from time to time. If you know in advance which restaurant you'll be dining at, visit its website; most restaurants now list nutritional information online. Planning your order in advance takes the guesswork out of restaurant meals and you won't have to flip through a menu full of tempting, high-fat options to select your dinner. If you can't find any nutritional information listed, consult generic calorie guides and use your best judgement. Contrary to popular belief, salads aren't always healthy – a bed of lettuce does not subtract calories from the cheese, dressing and fried meat in your salad. When in doubt, eat a light meal before you go and take apple cider vinegar. You may find that you're only hungry enough for an appetizer.

Skip the alcohol. As any college freshman quickly learns, alcohol is a weight gain monster. Ounce-for-ounce, hard alcohol is almost on par with melted butter for calorie content, and it provides absolutely no nutrients. To make matters worse, mixed drinks also contain sugary syrups that drive your insulin into overdrive. In the world of nutrition, alcohol is what's known as "empty calories"; they'll make you gain weight without gaining any benefit from having consumed them. If you must drink, restrict yourself to a single serving and stay away from hard liquor – light beer or red wine is a much more health-conscious choice.

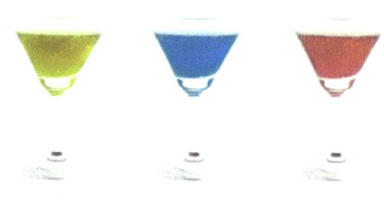

A single martini can have up to 330 calories.

Keep sweet treats in the freezer. Everyone craves chocolates or other goodies from time to time, but keeping those treats easily accessible can lead to overindulgence. Putting sweets in the freezer puts them out of sight and out of mind – if you have to wait for your treat to thaw out, you're less inclined to gorge yourself. Frozen chocolate also lasts longer in your mouth, so you don't need to eat as much. If you suffer from frequent chocolate cravings, consider keeping a bag of chocolate kisses in your freezer for a guilt-free indulgence.

Always start with water. It seems surprising for such a vital function, but the human body is incredibly bad at knowing when it's actually hungry. Hunger is the go-to response for when the body needs something, even if you're actually thirsty. When hunger pangs strike, start by drinking water and apple cider vinegar. Then wait fifteen minutes to see if you're actually hungry. You'll likely find that you aren't as ravenous as you were moments before.

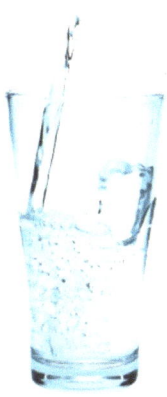

Drinking more water can improve a variety of health conditions.

Carry snacks with you at all times. It may seem counter-intuitive, but one thing that healthy, thin people have in common is that they are constantly eating. If you root through the purse of the healthiest person in your life, you're almost certain to find some sort of snack stowed away. Waiting for long periods of time between meals means you'll be starving by the time you next see food; you're much more likely to overeat. Snacking throughout the day keeps your blood sugar and metabolism constant, and it'll leave you more inclined to choose a light meal at dinner.

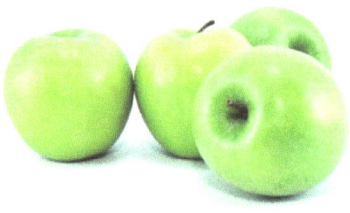

An apple a day can keep you from stuffing yourself in the evening.

Volunteer to bring the treats. Birthdays, potlucks and other social gatherings often involve tempting arrays of fat-loaded treats. How are you supposed to resist? Whenever possible, offer to contribute some baking of your own to a social event. Having a lower-calorie option available will let you join in without breaking your calorie limit.

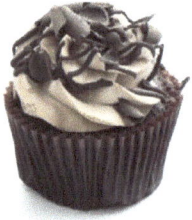

Well-meaning cupcakes are the bane of a dieting office worker's life.

Find low-calorie versions of your favorite recipes. Family favorite recipes are hard to part with, but they can be laden with fat and calories. Read up on low-calorie cooking substitutions – for instance, applesauce can be substituted for eggs, mashed cauliflower can replace mashed potatoes, and margarine can replace butter or shortening – to make your favorite meals a little easier on your waistline. Oftentimes, a massive reduction in calories only means a minor change in taste.

5 Tracking Progress

Staying motivated is one of the hardest parts of weight loss. As humans we like instant gratification for our actions; our caveman ancestors were instantly rewarded when they speared a deer, and we'd like to see pounds immediately fall off our bodies the minute we finish our garden salads. Unfortunately, as we all know, the world just doesn't work like that, and successful dieters must find ways to track their progress over time to keep morale up.

Obviously, stepping on a scale is the easiest way to keep track of your progression towards your goal. Weigh yourself once a week, and once a week only – daily weigh-ins can make you feel like you're treading water without making any progress. The ideal time to weigh yourself is first thing in the morning, as your stomach will be empty and there are fewer extraneous factors that could be influencing your weight. Try to do every weigh-in on the same bathroom scale; some scales are "lighter" or "heavier", but if you stick to the same one, you'll get an accurate measure of your total weight loss.

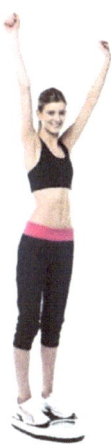

Getting on the scale won't always be a bad experience.

Numbers on the scale aren't the only way to tell that you're slimming down. On the first day of your new life, take a cloth tape measure and make a complete set of body measurements – measure your waist, hips, bust, and arm and thigh circumference. Keep them on a sheet of paper or on your computer somewhere, and take new measurements periodically. You may be surprised at the change. Numbers on the scale don't always correspond to a change in appearance. Water retention can wreak havoc with your numeric weight – a few days of salty foods can make it seems like you've packed on pounds overnight – while your body fat continues to drop. Taking measurements gives you a much more realistic sense of how your body is changing.

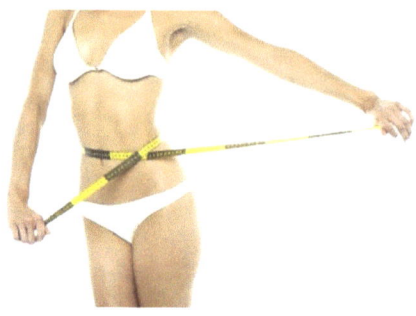

Waist measurements are a great indicator of health and size.

A fun way to track your progress is with photographs. You've probably seen hundreds of composite "before and after" shots, and creating your own is a great way to validate your hard work. Take a frontal shot and side view shot when you first start. Be honest – no sucking in your gut. Months later, when you've lost a significant amount of weight, repeat your photo shoot and put the sets of pictures side-by-side. It's tough to appreciate how much weight you're losing when it takes place so gradually. Keeping a picture log of your journey makes it clear how far you've come.

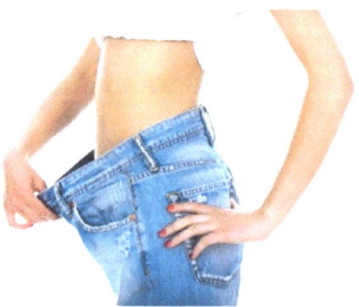

Visual proof of weight loss means more than any number on the scale.

If you're going to a gym regularly or using a personal trainer, you can also measure your progress by checking your percent body fat. A trainer will use a metal device that looks like a bit like a socket wrench to pinch your side and determine what portion of your body is actually blubber. As you burn off that fat and build up your muscle, that percentage will gradually go down. Getting an accurate measurement of your percent body fat may not be something you can do at home, but it's one of the most accurate ways to determining the improvement in your health.

Of course, many people on a weight loss journey find that their losses slow down and plateau. This is normal, and it shouldn't be a reason to panic. In the beginning, when you have lots of extra fat to lose, the shock of your new diet and exercise regime will have your body rapidly burning through the pounds. Once your body begins to acclimatize to your new lifestyle, naturally, progress will slow. This plateau period is the most dangerous time for someone aspiring to be healthy; it can feel like your efforts are pointless, and, in frustration, it may be tempting to return to your old bad habits.

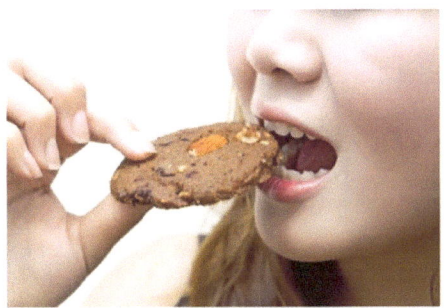

It's tough to justify avoiding unhealthy foods when your healthy lifestyle isn't producing results.

If you find yourself in a plateau, there are a few things you can do to keep yourself focused on progress. The obvious solution is to change up your routine; decrease your calorie limit and increase the frequency and intensity of your exercise regime. If you're still making very slow, gradual progress, you may want to spend some time focusing on how far you've already come. Buy yourself a whole new wardrobe – moving from ill-fitting clothing to all-new outfits will give you more self-confidence and make you feel like you're moving forward. Have a professional photo shoot to show off your new body. Treat yourself to a dress or suit that you dreamed of owning when you were larger.

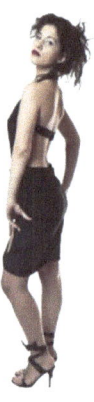

Nothing boosts confidence like new, flattering clothes.

Through your entire progression – no matter how you're tracking your weight loss – it's most important to set and strive for goals. Having an overall goal – such as losing 80lbs – is noble, but it can be intimidating when you're starting your journey. Set little goals along the way and work for them. Most people agree that losing 5lbs isn't difficult; make yourself a chain of small goals and milestones that will get you down to your ideal. So long as you stay focused on your objective and remain dedicated to a healthy lifestyle, you'll meet your goals in the long run – no matter how slowly you go.

6 What to Do When Nothing Works

Sometimes, despite our best efforts, weight loss just doesn't happen. You have a tough time sticking to your diet and exercise regime, or you may be trying your hardest and not seeing results. If you're stuck in a rut, there are place to turn to kick-start your weight loss.

The first person you should speak to if your weight loss program isn't working is your doctor. You may have an underlying condition – like an untreated thyroid problem – that is preventing you from losing weight. You doctor can check you for any problems, and give you tips or resources that can quickly correct the problem.

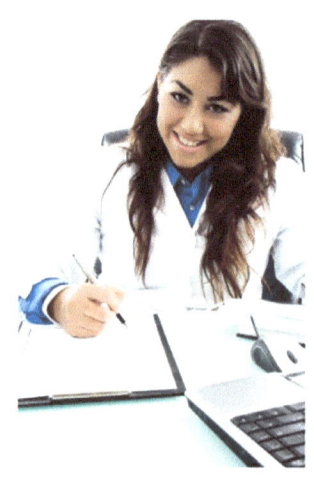

Always check with your doctor before starting a new weight loss plan.

If sticking to your diet is an issue, your first step should be to increase your daily intake of apple cider vinegar. There is a direct relationship between the amount of vinegar you take and how full you feel; if you take doses of vinegar throughout the day, you should be able to maintain your resolve from sunup to sundown.

Another method of tackling diet-related problems is to see a dietician. You should be able to find one online or in your local yellow pages. Keep a detailed food diary for a few days prior to your appointment, noting the times, quantities and types of food you eat. Your dietician can use this information to offer you suggestions for improving your diet and kick-starting your weight loss. You may even be able to work with your dietician to come up with healthy meal plans to get you through your week.

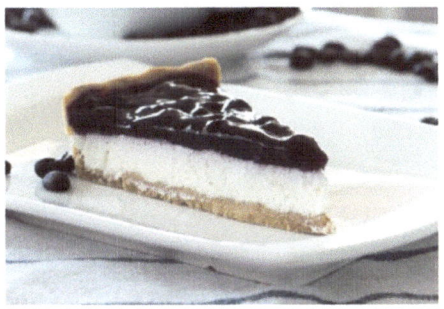

It's important to be honest with your dietician, no matter what you've eaten.

If you haven't already, you should consider hiring a personal trainer. Even a few sessions with a trainer can give you a better idea of where your fitness is at, and the trainer can help you design a personalized exercise program to follow after you've stopped paying for sessions. If money is tight, many trainers will offer small group sessions for you and a friend or two, which gets you personalized attention at a fraction of the cost.

If stress-eating or emotional eating are known problems for you, your best source of help isn't going to be in a gym or a dietician's office – you should seek out a psychologist. For many people, weight gain isn't the result of carelessness or greed; instead, it has its roots in emotional triggers and un-dealt-with issues. Some psychologists specialize in obesity and emotional eating, and they can help you get through the problems you need to conquer before any real weight loss can begin. The cost of seeing a psychologist may be steep, but you'll save yourself a lot of time, frustration and heartache.

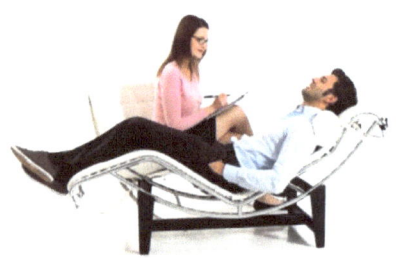

Undiagnosed psychological disorders can also be obstacles to weight loss.

If you live with a family, your nearest and dearest loved ones may be the source of your failure. It's tough to nibble on garden salad while your family wolfs down pizza, and preparing separate meals every night is a pain. Talk to your family about getting on board with your healthy lifestyle. You need their support if you're going to succeed, and the entire family will be healthier for it. Changing the family diet might be tough, at first, but getting the entire family out to exercise together might be a good way to start.

Another culprit may be an over-packed schedule. It's a simple fact: it's a lot quicker and easier to pop a burrito in the microwave than it is to roast a chicken breast. If you're the kind of person who's constantly on the go, plan ahead. Make meals in advance and package them for easy microwaving. Brown-bag a lunch, and spare yourself the calories of a fast-food midday meal. Eating better will actually increase your energy, making your daily rush easier to handle. here

7 Apple Cider Vinegar Recipes

Apple cider vinegar has some incredible properties, but there is one drawback – you have to actually put it in your mouth. This form of vinegar has a much stronger odor and taste than the white and malt vinegars you may be used to, and some find the distinct flavor unpleasant. There's no need to panic if you cringe at the thought of eating vinegar-soaked bread; there are plenty of other alternatives that nicely disguise the flavor.

You probably wouldn't want to suck back a glass of plain apple cider vinegar through a straw, but you can use it to make a delightful, chilled beverage. Put your apple cider vinegar in the fridge; when it's cold, mix half a cup of it with two cups of water and a quarter of a cup of organic grape juice. You can add more grape juice if the drink tastes too sour for you at the end. Add a tablespoon of lemon juice, then stir in a teaspoon of organic honey and half a teaspoon of powdered cinnamon. Stir the drink until all ingredients are well-mixed, and serve with ice cubes. In addition to fighting fat, some claim that this drink will also fight hangovers.

You can also use apple cider vinegar to make a delightful vinaigrette salad dressing. Stir two tablespoons of Dijon mustard, one third of a cup of lemon juice, half a teaspoon of curry powder and a handful of chopped chives into a cup of apple cider vinegar. Whisk in three quarters of a cup of olive oil. Be sure to shake this dressing will before adding it to your salad.

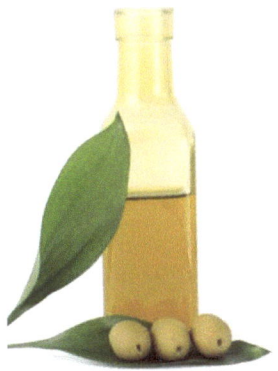

Extra virgin olive oil is the best choice for homemade salad dressing.

Apple cider vinegar can also be hidden in a variety of canned and homemade soups. Creamy, dense soups work best. Gradually add vinegar to your soup until you begin to taste it, and enjoy. Individual preferences vary. Some people report that apple cider vinegar goes nicely into root-vegetable-based soups; soups that contain beets, parsnips or sweet potatoes will do nicely. It also adds a pleasant kick to lentil soups.

The sharp, tangy flavor of apple cider vinegar also makes it well-suited for use in baked beans and sweet potato recipes. You can add a touch of vinegar into your favorite baked bean recipe – stir in vinegar one tablespoon at a time, tasting after each addition. You can also drizzle apple cider vinegar over peeled sweet potatoes before baking them in the oven. Some people have even successfully incorporated the vinegar into braised cabbage recipes.

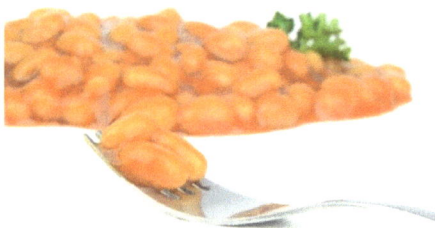

Use vinegar to add zest to your beans and make them more filling.

In place of soy sauce, apple cider vinegar can also be used to spice up boiled rice and grains. Soy sauce is chock-full of sodium, making vinegar a healthier alternative. You can try it on quinoa, flax, Jerusalem couscous, barley, rye and wild rice.

Ultimately, you're free to be adventurous and experiment. You can substitute in apple cider vinegar for other varieties of vinegar in your recipes. Use it on salads, meats, grains, fish and sauces. It doesn't matter how you choose to take the vinegar, so long as you're getting some every day.

Conclusion

With a proper combination of careful eating, plentiful exercise and apple cider vinegar, your weight loss goals are easily reachable. Be patient, and stay focused – all it takes a little bit of determination. Calorie counting and exercise alone will take off pounds, but apple cider vinegar is a key component for making the process painless. Not only will your blood sugar stabilize and your blood pressure lower, but the appetite-suppression properties of apple cider vinegar will protect you from the hunger pangs that plague most dieting hopefuls.

No matter your goal – if you have ten pounds to lose or one hundred – this apple cider weight loss plan can help. Get out your measuring tape and camera, and prepare to be amazed by your transformation. Your health will improve, your energy will increase, and, best of all, your old jeans will finally fit again.

Just don't forget to stock up on vinegar.

ABOUT THE AUTHOR

Melody McAdams was born and raised in Pasco, Washington and worked for her uncle Rudy picking apples. She is a certified weight loss nutritionist and has used Apple Cider Vinegar for years, not only in her own life, but recommends it for her clients. Melody now lives in Macon, Georgia and works as a health coach.